Getting Rid
of
FIBROIDS

by

Deborah Bellis Khalidi

ISBN 978-1-300-61853-9

INTRODUCTION

It is my sincerest wish that each and every female reader that has been diagnosed with troublesome fibroids will take a positive stance in their determination to seek, as far as is able – peace with themselves and those around them. At first glance, this may seem a rather odd statement to make in a book containing facts and information about fibroids and gynaecological health and already I can hear some of you saying "it is easier said than done". I agree, not only from my experience as a holistic therapist and counsellor, but also from my own personal experience and as having been diagnosed with problematic fibroids. However, it is my hope that as the reader progresses through this book, that they will come to understand, if not already, the relevance of the above statement concerned with that of finding peace with oneself and with others and that connected to the subject of fibroids. To make this more clear; apart from the physiological and biological aspects and so forth concerned with that of fibroids and of which is readily discussed in this book, we shall also see, as it is being increasingly recognised today, that the emotional factors in our lives, past and present, are a major contribution to the development of problematic fibroids.

And so with great understanding of the suffering that is brought to the individual through this often debilitating condition, I dedicate therefore this book to all my sisters around the world who have battled and/or is still battling with problematic fibroids and the complications and anxieties that come with the diagnosis - fear of infertility, miscarriage, loss of the womb, hospital procedures and the agonising decisions that one is ultimately faced with when one is diagnosed with one or more problematic fibroids. Indeed, I heard one lady describe her fibroids as being like "gremlins in the womb" and I am sure that other fibroid sufferers would readily agree, for they can seem to spring up overnight and are a menace, causing considerable distress and discomfort to the unfortunate sufferer.

I have aimed to give hope and informative positive advice in this book, as all aspects are considered including the treatment of fibroids via allopathic medicine and surgery and also via the many wonderful, natural and alternative therapies that are available today. Lifestyle and diet is also examined. However, and most importantly, the need for the consideration of the emotional and spiritual aspects are looked at in great depth and in relation to its relevance concerning fibroids and gynaecological conditions in general. Our emotional state can greatly contribute to sickness and disease and in particular to that of fibroids and gynaecological health in women.

My appreciation, thanks and well wishes goes out to all those who have taken the step to buy this book. I am deeply honoured and grateful and hope it serves you well, my friend.

Your friend, Deborah Bellis Khalidi.

INDEX

Chapter 1
Fibroids – What are they?

Chapter 2
Looking at the importance of Diet and Vitamins for the treatment of fibroids

Chapter 3
Looking at Alternative Therapies for the treatment of fibroids

Chapter 4 The emotional factor and its contribution to the development of fibroids

Chapter 1

What are fibroids?

"...I'm always having to pass water frequently and then there is never any real feeling of total relief...I'm often up several times in the night and often exhausted the next day...."

".....It's extremely uncomfortable...lower back problems, bloating and the awful cramping and I get pretty fed up with people asking if I'm pregnant because of the abnormal size of my uterus..."

"...I constantly feel drained from the heavy bleeding and often dread leaving

*the house for fear I'm going to have
another awful episode of extreme
gushing...It is very restricting and
debilitating...."*

If the above statements seem to ring an
all too familiar bell to you then you are
probably one of the many women who
have been diagnosed with and/or are
suffering with the common symptoms
of fibroids. But what are fibroids?

Fibroids are very common. They are
the most common female, benign
tumour of the pelvic organs. That
means that they are not malignant or
sinister or cancerous, but they are
growths of the muscle of the womb
wall. Fibroids are benign growths of
the muscular wall of the uterus
therefore, and so can be in various

different sites in the uterus. Depending on where they are, they are named differently. So if they are within the womb cavity, protruding out from the lining of the womb they are called sub-mucous fibroids. If they are in the wall of the uterus they are called intramural (inside the wall) and if they are on the external surface of the uterus they are called serosal. Then there is another type of fibroid that is called pedunculated and that means it is on the outside of the uterine wall and it is attached to the outside of the wall by a stalk, a peduncle. So there are lots of different types of uterine fibroids and these names describe their geographical location.

Symptoms that a person may have with fibroids

There are lots of different symptoms that fibroids may give rise to and it is important to say that you may not know that you have got a fibroid or fibroids because some women have no symptoms at all. Of course there is the question, why do some women have symptoms; period problems, pain, fertility problems, all sorts of things, (we will come back to that later) whereas others seem to manage to get away with it and only have their fibroids diagnosed by accident, because they are having, for example, a family planning appointment or a smear done or an ultrasound scan for something totally different. The other interesting thing about fibroids is that you would expect the biggest fibroids to cause the most problems and the little fibroids not to, but unfortunately they are a law unto themselves. Apparently there are women with very small fibroids who are debilitated by pain or who cannot get pregnant or are miscarrying. Other women with massive fibroids are sailing through with no complications at all.

In general terms those that are on the outside surface are much less likely to cause period problems or problems getting pregnant for example, whereas, if you have got fibroids in the cavity it can then be understand that this might lead to heavy bleeding or pain, or problems with an embryo implanting. However, and as mentioned previously, fibroids follow no rules and apparently, the more there is to learn about them, the more there is the increasing realization, especially in the medical world, that there is a lot more left to learn.

The range of treatments available for people diagnosed with fibroids

There are lots of treatments for fibroids and it very much depends on the presenting symptoms and as to what is going to be the most suitable treatment. There are surgical treatments to remove them and these can be open surgical procedures like a myomectomy or even a hysterectomy for women who are at the end of their reproductive life. There are laparoscopic or key-hole procedures to remove them and of course there are the newer, minimally invasive treatments, some of which for example, are being pioneered in hospitals within the U.K. and other parts of the world. Indeed, the latest minimally invasive treatments do not even require the insertion of a telescope, the procedure being performed by inserting laser fibres or the most recent by focused ultrasound. This is done under a magnetic resonance scanner. The patient is put into the scanner and basically, high intensity ultrasound beams are shone at the fibroids, focusing them into the fibroid. They heat the fibroid up and the fibroid dies and shrinks in size. This is a very pioneering and innovative treatment for women with fibroids but especially for those women who are having repeated miscarriages or having problems getting pregnant as this form of treatment helps to preserve their fertility whilst treating the fibroid or fibroids and without subjecting them to surgery which may lead to subsequent sub-fertility. For example, although a myomectomy is a wonderful operation and is often recommended particularly for very big fibroids, a myomectomy comes with the risk of scar tissue developing which can compromise a woman's ability to get pregnant in the future. This is an important point for the medical person to consider before he or she commits a woman who is trying to have a baby or trying to get pregnant in the future, to fibroid surgery.

Besides surgery and the above mentioned imaging techniques there are of course drugs. There are many types of drugs such as hormonal treatments that can be used. For example the combined oral contraceptive pill can be helpful for women who present with heavy bleeding. There are drugs called gonadotrophin releasing hormones (GnRH) which tells the brain to shut down the menstrual cycle and stop all hormones going to the ovaries so you do become pseudo-menopausal while you are taking these drugs. The symptoms are reversible but while taking the GnRH you get hot flushes and other menopausal symptoms because the cycle is cancelled. There are all sorts of new medicines that are being trialled at the moment, for example progesterone modulators. However, in general, these medical treatments are recognised by the medical practitioner as being more of a stop gap or interim measure and if you need a definite treatment you are usually going to have to pursue some form of surgical procedure or one of the new themal ablation minimally invasive techniques.

In view of the above, we can see that some of the medical treatments mentioned may not be suitable for women that are trying to get pregnant based on the fact that they may or can stop the cycle. The last thing that is needed if you are trying to get pregnant is to take drugs that stop your natural cycle and prevent ovulation, and experience menopausal symptoms even though these side effects are all reversible. However, there are occasions when a short sharp burst of medical therapy before the woman tries to get pregnant has been seen to be helpful.

The important thing about fibroids is that the physician or doctor should not take a rigid view about what is the best treatment for a particular type of fibroid. What really matters is that the medical practitioner should work out the priority list for what the patient wants to resolve together. For example, and in this case, the doctor can ask the patient to tell him/her which symptom is at the top of the priority list. The doctor could then ask, if there is one symptom he could sort out, which one would it be? This would be good practise as sometimes treating the bleeding and the pain or the pressure on her bladder is incompatible with the fact that the female patient wants a baby. Similarly, if she has completed her family, then possibly the woman may choose to get rid of the offending fibroid and the entire uterus that goes with it, so she does not have any further problems. In this case there are no rigid rules on how this fibroid should be treated by that treatment. It is really important that the woman is looked at holistically, (and really this is the point of this book) so that together the best option can be found available for her.

In looking at this fact briefly and the importance of the holistic well being of the patient (we shall be looking at non-medical or alternative treatments in depth, a little further on) some women have experimented with Chinese herbal medicines and acupuncture and homeopathy and there are a variety of products that are available on the internet and websites that claim to be treatments for fibroids. Many women are enthusiastic about them and my belief is also that until conventional medicine has found a solution to every problem then the door should not be shut on alternative medicines.

How fibroids can affect women's fertility

Fibroids can have an adverse affect on fertility (the ability to get pregnant) but predominantly due to where they are located in the uterus. So, for example, if you have got fibroids inside the cavity, you can understand how it might be difficult for an embryo to implant because they may well have changed the physical or hormonal environment there. Or they may indeed be producing chemicals that are adverse to implantation. However, although I have mentioned that fibroids on the outside surface of the uterus are less likely to affect your fertility, they may still affect it if they are for example positioned beside a fallopian tube and blocking or pressing upon it and that might well be a problem. It is really very individualised. As mentioned earlier, some women with tiny fibroids have endless problems with fertility and women with massive fibroids have uncomplicated pregnancies. Fibroids are a law unto themselves.

Statistics show that Afro-Caribbean women are more commonly affected by fibroids

As yet, it is not understood in the medical field why afro-Caribbean women are more commonly affected by fibroids although it has been recognised that there must be some sort of genetic predisposition because they are more common in Afro-Caribbean women and in these women they also occur at a younger age.

Fibroids in general are terribly common and it is important to get this into perspective. They are so common that it is thought as many as 40-50% of women will have fibroids, not all of which may be symptomatic. On the basis of post-mortem studies, there are masses of women who have got fibroids in the uterus and many of them, if you ask their families may not have had any complaints. However, they are so common and they are a very important reason for women to seek gynaecological help. Some 20% of all gynaecological outpatient appointments are apparently fibroid related which is a huge number!

1 in 5 women coming to routine gynaecological outpatients will be there because of a symptom from their fibroids. Probably the most common symptom that fibroids cause is heavy periods. They can be torrentially heavy with fibroids. A woman may describe hers as being like a pouring tap or passing large clots, often flooding at night and not being able to go out of the front door because she is so frightened of having an uncontrollable and embarrassing accident in a public place. Some women are literally padded up as if the have got nappies on, because they cannot predict the extent of the flow. This is a dreadful imposition on a lifestyle if you cannot go out of the door every month of your

life and cannot go to work. So, period problems are one of the major symptoms that women with fibroids are likely to suffer from as well as pressure symptoms. If the fibroids is pressing on your bladder or your bowel it can be very uncomfortable and very painful, and we have already discussed how a large mass can have an adverse affect on fertility. When a woman gets pregnant there are all sorts of things that could happen. First and foremost they may have no problems; the fibroid may just sit there in the uterus. It may get bigger because it is stimulated by the hormones of pregnancy to enlarge but it may not cause problems. On the other hand, it can be the cause of early miscarriages and late miscarriages and therefore something very specific to pregnancy called red degeneration. This is when the woman presents classically at about 20/22 weeks with very severe abdominal pain. Often deciding whether she has problems with the flood or an acute appendix can be difficult. What has happened is that the dramatic or rapid growth in the size of the fibroid due to the stimulus of the pregnancy hormones, has meant that the fibroid has almost outgrown its own blood supply and the centre of it dies, necroses, undergoes cell death and that degenerates and causes the release of very painful chemicals or cytokines from the fibroid which cause the pain. This sort of situation can or may affect the pregnancy adversely.

The patient hopefully can be given pain relief and things may quieten down. However, what can happen is that the acute episode in the fibroid can stimulate the uterus to start contracting and might possibly therefore, cause the woman to go into premature labour and depending on how many weeks she is it would be classified as a late miscarriage or an early pre-term delivery/possible neo-natal death.

Fibroids can cause problems at the time of the delivery. If the fibroid is in the way of the baby's head descending into the birth canal that is going to be a problem and there may be the need for a caesarean section. A caesarean section for a woman who is not able to deliver the baby because the passage of the baby is being blocked by the fibroid is likely to be more difficult because after cutting through fibroid tissue in order to deliver the baby it can be quite difficult to stop the bleeding from those fibroids when repairing the uterine muscle again. On a lighter note and a point which must be emphasised, is that there are lots of women with fibroids who have pregnancies that are successful too.

It is important that if you think you have fibroids that you seek advice. If you have painful periods, heavy periods, abdominal pain or you find that you have got an enlarged uterus, ask for help. Sometimes women visit the doctor saying that they have not got any of these symptoms but that they have got a lump and of course they are terrified that it is something sinister. Your doctor, in this case, will probably organise for you to have an examination. Most general practitioners will be able to identify that the uterus is enlarged and they will probably organise for you to have an ultrasound scan and you can then start the dialogue about how to manage your fibroid. It may well be that you don't need to have any treatment at all because you may not have symptoms that are troublesome. In this case, the doctor will most likely reassure you that the lump that you sometimes feel lying down in the morning in bed is actually quite benign and is a fibroid and so you may not require anything further in the way of conventional treatment and/ or surgery. On the other hand, you may be one of the unfortunate women who have suffered from debilitating heavy, painful periods for many years but just thought that you had to put up with it and that that was something you had to accept and part of being a woman. However, and on the contrary, you need to be reassured that there is something that can be done to make you feel a lot better.

CHAPTER 2
Looking at the importance of diet and vitamins when treating fibroids

Many women seek out alternative ways of treating fibroids rather than opting for surgery and one way that women can help themselves is by looking at foods that shrink fibroids. Although diet on its own will not get rid of fibroids, there is no doubt that diet is an extremely important part of your overall strategy should you wish to use natural treatments.

Maintaining a healthy diet is crucial to overall health when diagnosed with a fibroid tumour. One of the most important principles to remember is that you should stick with the components of a general healthy diet whether you have fibroids or not.

However, there are specific elements you should both include and exclude to give you the best chance of seeing an improvement.

The first thing you should do is ensure that you are well hydrated. Drinking plenty of water ensures that toxins are flushed out of the body and if you do not drink enough fluids, toxins will accumulate in the organs, and this is thought to be one of the various reasons why fibroids form. In addition, constipation can be a by-product of not drinking enough and this again causes the accumulation of waste products which can be reabsorbed into the body.

With regard to a fibroid diet, you should firstly ensure that you buy organic foods wherever possible. The bulk of your general diet should consist of grains, fresh fruits and vegetables seeds nuts and essential oils. Meats should form a small part of your diet and you should avoid eating any processed meats, such as sausages and salami, and fatty meats.

Fresh fruits are loaded with vitamins and bioflavonoid which are excellent for the body. Rather than concentrating on which fresh fruits you eat, it is important to understand, that they are all beneficial and to thoroughly wash the exterior of fruits and eat the skins where possible. Obviously some are better for you than others as they contain concentrated nutrients, such as kiwi fruits and blueberries but on the whole, a good balance of as wide a range of fruits is the best approach.

Other foods that shrink fibroids are vegetables. As with fruits, a balanced approach is best. Nutrients are generally higher when foods are in their raw state so get into the habit of eating a salad daily, made up of a 'rainbow' of coloured vegetables as in general, the brighter the colour, the higher the nutrients. If you cook vegetables, ensure they are just lightly cooked – steaming is an excellent way to preserve water soluble nutrients. If you do cook them in water, try to use the water in gravies or sauces.

Onions and garlic deserve a special mention. They are both excellent sources of antioxidants and help keep your female hormones in balance. You should include them wherever possible, particularly in their raw form.

Eating the correct oils is also important for a fibroid diet. Olive oil and the Omega oils contained in oily fish are particularly useful for the body. Avoid saturated fats, including butters and those in cheeses.

With regard to meats, try to stick to fish and lean white meat such as chicken, choosing organic where possible. If you do eat red meats, stick to very lean cuts from a reputable source. It is also worth trying soya burgers and vegetarian 'sausages' if you enjoy these types of foods.

Other foods that shrink fibroids include beans, nuts and seeds, the most beneficial being flax, pumpkin and sunflower.

Weight – a contributing factor in the risk of uterine fibroids

It is important to understand that on their own, foods that shrink fibroids will not be as effective when the dietary element is thought of as just one part of an overall treatment strategy for fibroids. Not only is diet important, but you will need to make lifestyle changes if you want to see significant success.

One factor proven to increase the risk of uterine fibroids is obesity. The result of a study published in a 1991 issue of Nutrition suggested uterine fibroids that present with symptoms may be associated with obesity.

This was given further credence in a study published in a 1998 issue of Epidemiology, which showed evidence those women with body mass index above 30 experienced a 23 percent greater chance of developing uterine fibroids.

The importance of vitamins in the treatment of fibroids

We have looked at the importance of a diet rich in vitamins for shrinking fibroids and to restore the health of your reproductive system. However, it is also important to consult a medical professional before treating fibroids with vitamin supplements.

Vitamin C

Vitamin C is a water-soluble antioxidant that strengthens the immune system and protects the body from infections, viruses and diseases that can cause fibroid tumours. Vitamin C also relieves fibroid-related menstrual pain and cramps, eases heavy menstrual bleeding, reduces uterine inflammation that can worsen fibroid symptoms, prevents fibroid tumour growth by regulating oestrogen levels and helps fibroid tumours heal. The recommended daily dosage for vitamin C is 1,000mg for women. Foods rich in vitamin C include strawberries, cranberries, blueberries, tomatoes, broccoli, spinach, Swiss chard, kale, oranges, lemons, pineapples, kiwi and grapefruit.

Vitamin D

Vitamin D is a fat-soluble vitamin that aids in calcium absorption, reduces inflammation, eases menstrual pain, shrinks fibroids, supports a healthy reproductive system, repairs damaged tissues, relieves cramping, heals wounds and improves uterine muscle tone. The recommended daily dosage for vitamin D is 15mcg for women. Foods rich in vitamin D include cod liver oil, salmon, mushrooms, mackerel, fortified yogurt, eggs, swiss cheese, beef liver, fortified milk and fortified orange juice.

Vitamin E

Vitamin E is a fat-soluble antioxidant that improves immune system function and protects your body from damaging free radicals that can cause or worsen fibroid tumours. Vitamin E also heals wounds, reduces inflammation, repairs damaged tissues, eases cramping and relieves menstrual pain. The recommended daily dosage for vitamin E is 15mg for women. Foods rich in vitamin E include almonds, broccoli, peanut butter, pecans, avocados, spinach, sunflower seeds, and soybean oil. Kiwi, mangoes, corn oil and tomatoes.

Vitamin K

Vitamin K is a fat-soluble vitamin that aids in blood clot formation, reduces heavy bleeding, regulates cellular growth, shrinks fibroids and eases menstrual cramps. The recommended daily dosage for vitamin K is 90 mcg for women. Foods rich in vitamin K include Romaine lettuce, cabbage, broccoli, kale, yogurt, kefir, egg yolks, soy products, pears, strawberries and papayas.

Diet plan for shrinking and treating fibroids

A few changes in your daily diet can help to prevent the development of fibroids and shrink existing fibroids. For this diet plan you will need:

Black molasses
Milk
Vitamin supplement with iron
Apple cider vinegar
Nattokinase soy beans
Tofu
Pinto beans
Black beans
Kidney beans

Fresh vegetables
Fruits
Low-fat dairy products

1. Mix 2 tbsp. molasses with 6 oz. milk and 1 tsp. water in a glass. Drink the concoction two times a day to improve internal iron levels, remedy issues related to anaemia and increase your potassium intake.

2. Drink 2 tsp. apple cider vinegar mixed with 8 oz. of water once a day to help with fat loss, and to purify the body of toxins.

3. Eat one serving of nattokinase soy beans every day to help shrink fibroid tissue. Add one vitamin supplement with iron to your daily diet to improve iron levels and resupply your body with vital vitamins and minerals.

4. Eat tofu three times a week to help lower your levels of oestrogen.

5. Incorporate pinto beans, split peas, lima beans, black beans and kidney beans into your diet to diminish oestrogen levels and thwart fibroid growth. Eat at least one helping of beans every day.

6. Eliminate meats from your diet and increase your intake of fresh fruit and vegetables to keep oestrogen levels down.

7. Avoid high-fat milk and cheeses. Incorporate low-fat dairy products into your diet to keep oestrogen levels down.

8. Incorporate a serving of fish into your diet at least three times a week.

Include helpings of salmon, mackerel, cold-water fish and tuna to reduce inflamed tissues and fibroid irritation.

The negatives of some dairy products

Look for alternatives when buying substitutes for dairy; such as low-fat, organic products, or omega-rich foods. Dairy products contain calcium, which is important, so when removing the high fat dairy products, try these foods still rich in calcium; soybeans, bean, peas, soy milk, goats milk, nut milk, sesame seeds, and green leafy vegetables. These foods easily pass through the liver, which results in less oestrogen in the body. The more oestrogen in the body, the higher the risk for fibroid tumours or aggravating current tumours.

Caffeinated Beverages and Alcohol are Bad

Alcohol is a major toxin to the liver. Alcohol prevents the liver from performing properly. If the liver isn't functioning properly, it will not metabolize hormones. This will lead to

increasing oestrogen levels, which is bad for fibroid tumour. Also causing the same problem as alcohol are caffeinated beverages, as well as drinks like fruit juices and sodas containing large amounts of sugar. Consume drinks that are caffeine free, low in sugar and without alcohol. Water is the best thing you can drink.

CHAPTER 3

LOOKING AT ALTERNATIVE THERAPIES IN THE TREATMENT OF FIBROIDS

Herbal Medicine and its use in the treatment of fibroids

Herbal remedies to shrink fibroids have been used for many years, particularly by Chinese doctors. There is a strong interest in using natural remedies to treat fibroids as more and more women are turning their backs on invasive surgery. Herbal medicine – also called botanical medicine or phytomedicine – refers to using a plant's seeds, berries, roots, leaves, bark, or flowers of medicinal purposes. Herbalism has a long tradition of use outside of conventional medicine. It is becoming more mainstream as improvements in analysis and quality control along with advances in clinical research show the value of herbal medicine in the treating and preventing disease.

Herbal remedies for fibroids are not usually successful when used in isolation, although you will see herbal preparations being sold from various sources which claim that they will shrink fibroids. Having said this, there is no doubt whatsoever that they can form an extremely valuable part of a comprehensive treatment for fibroids, particularly where symptomatic relief is concerned. In addition, herbs for fibroids are incorporated in many plans which involve liver detoxing, as it is well known that for some women, their fibroids probably stem from a build up of environmental toxins which are licked inside the liver, wreaking havoc.

One thing to bear in mind is that although herbs are natural, in certain quantities and combinations, they can be potent and can cause serious harm if taken in the wrong quantities. As far as treating fibroids is concerned, you can often buy ready-made preparations which have the correct, safe dosages stated on the labels.

The herbs which are commonly used for treating fibroids include:-

Milk Thistle
Dandelion Root
Artichoke Extract
Yam
Ginger
Willow
Cinnamon

In regards to the treatment of fibroids, the herbal remedies are reported to slowly reduce the size of fibroids and control the further growth of new ones, thus preventing the occurrence of complications caused by fibroids such as urinary problems, dysmenorrhoea, anaemia due to prolonged heavy bleeding and other symptoms associated with it. Many of the herbs and natural treatments look to reduce the effect of symptoms from fibroids, along with helping to balance the female reproductive system. It is believed that fibroids form due to an excess of oestrogen in the system. This is a particular problem just before the onset of menopause during the time called the perimenopause. Oestrogen levels can become extremely high during this time and if not properly balanced, can lead to the formation and growth of fibroid tumours. A key consideration in treating fibroids and encouraging their reduction is to treat the functioning of the liver. The liver acts as the main filter in the body, and helping it to remove toxins, may in fact help to rectify the excess levels of oestrogen in the body. This balance can be aided with the use of natural remedies such as and along with herbal preparations.

Herbal remedies can also attack fibroid tumours by working to increase progesterone levels in the body, thereby balancing the excess levels of oestrogen. If you are plagued with symptoms from fibroids like heavy bleeding, pain, cramping, bloating and fatigue; herbal teas and supplements may offer a solution.

Liver Cleanse

There are many formulations you can use to do a general liver cleanse. Specific herbs can target the liver, helping it to function more efficiently, reducing the level of oestrogen in the body. Liver friendly herbs like burdock, dandelion, yellow dock, red clover, nettle, cleavers, milk thistle and vervain, bump up hormone processing. Try combining equal parts of these herbs in one quart of boiling water. Steep for about ten minutes, strain and drink. Try using this remedy for 4 weeks, and take one week. Have your physician check your progress, and resume treatment if desired.

Chaste berry

Vitex, or chaste berry is a popular herbal treatment used to treat menstrual problems by raising levels of progesterone in the body. Instead of working as a phytoestrogen, vitex works on the hypothalamus and pituitary glands and balances the female hormones. By doing so, this can lead to a reduction in symptoms associated with fibroids, such as heavy bleeding, pressure and pain. Vitex or chaste berry is widely available in tea form or supplement form. Often it is combined with other beneficial herbs such as raspberry, which has also been shown to be of benefit to the female system. Follow dosing instructions carefully. Vitex is safe to consume indefinitely.

Castor Oil

Soothing castor oil packs are a good choice when it comes to treating fibroids. Thought to penetrate the internal organs, castor oil packs can be applied directly to the abdomen and may help shrink smaller fibroid tumours. Make a pack by saturating a small piece of flannel or cotton in some castor oil. Wring out well. Warm in the microwave for just a few seconds and place over the affected area. Cover with plastic wrap and top with a hot water bottle. Recline and relax for up to one hour. Repeat once a day for relief.

Consult your physician if you are having severe symptoms with your fibroids including extremely heavy cramping or bleeding, or pressure on internal organs. You may need more conventional treatment.

Homeopathy and its use in the treatment of fibroids

Homeopathy is a system of medicine which involves treating the individual with highly diluted substances, given mainly in tablet form with the aim of triggering the body's natural system of healing. Based on their specific symptoms, a homeopath will match the most appropriate medicine to each patient.

Homeopathy is based on the principle that you can treat 'like with like', that is, a substance which causes symptoms when taken in large doses, can be used in small amounts to treat those same symptoms. For example, drinking too much coffee can cause sleeplessness and agitation, so according to this principle, when made into a homeopathic medicine, it could be used to treat people with these symptoms. This concept is sometimes used to treat patients with ADHD, or small doses of allergens such as pollen are sometimes used to de-sensitise allergic patients. However, one major difference with homeopathic medicines is that substances are used in ultra high dilutions, which makes them non-toxic.

Surgery for fibroids can be a painful and risky way of removing uterine fibroids and one which, for example, the homeopathic practitioner would say that it can never work on the reoccurrence of these fibroids in the future. Homeopathy, they claim, is the safe, economical and side affect free way of getting rid of uterine fibroids. Not only does homeopathy remove the uterine fibroids without any risk but also stops them from reoccurrence, as after getting rid of uterine fibroids through homeopathy, the doctor prescribes a follow up course which stops the unwanted growth in the uterine area. Through the help of homeopathy and energy healing one can melt these fibroids within and let them pass away through the urine track. Therefore, according to the homeopathic practitioner, such a miracle is still not possible if you are going with allopathic treatments.

Homeopathy treats the uterine fibroids in a non invasive manner. The remedy homeopathy has to treat uterine fibroids is Silicae which behaves as a homeopathical scalpel. On the other hand another remedy for the same is Myrristica Sebifera. This in simpler terms is known as the homeopathical knife. The person suffering from fibroids is supposed to take both of these potions together which results in separation of the uterine fibroids from the uterus wall and then these tumours simply fall off. The homeopath has the remedy to export out the uterine fibroids present within. There are prescriptions in homeopathy which are helpful in letting the uterine fibroids export. Homeopaths according to individual reading, prescribe doses of Hepar Sulphuris Calcarea which is meant to catalyze the uterine fibroid growth. This prescription is combined with Myrristica and Silicae which works on exporting out the unwanted tissues.

Thus homeopathy is definitely suggested in uterine fibroids or myomas. While on homeopathic treatment the woman avoids surgical operation thus continuing their household and professional activities and saving money because it is well known that surgery leads to physical, mental, emotional and financial trauma. Homeopathy treatment under a competent homeopathic doctor may take time but it will avoid all the unwanted complications and will preserve the fertility of the female.

Moreover, even if surgery is chosen, homeopathic treatment is highly affective to prevent the formation of adhesions (scar tissue), which is a frequent sequel of myomectomy and hysterectomy.

There are 93 homeopathy medicines which give great relief in uterine fibroid or myoma. However, the correct choice and the resulting relief is a matter of experience and right judgment on the part of the homeopathic doctor. The treatment is decided after thorough case taking of the patient. Thus homeopathic remedies of uterine myomas or fibroids are tailor made unlike allopathy in which all patients receive the same drugs i.e. hormonal pills although trade name may be different.

Some of the homeopathic remedies which may be used in a case of uterine fibroid or myoma under an expert homeopathy doctor are Conium maculatum, Hydrastis, Hydrocotyle, Acid nitricum, Thuja occidantalis, Trillium pendulum, Thlaspi bursa, Aurum metallicum, Caulophyllum, Lachesis and so on.

For example, Aurum metallicum is used in cases with large fibroids, often prolapsing into vagina, associated with a deep sense of depression and hopelessness. Caulophyllum is used in patients with heavy bleeding with labour like cramps and passage of tissue with clots.

Thus homeopathy acts as a safe, effective, natural alternative to drugs, hormones and surgery. This is one of the diseases where homeopathy has been very effective in preventing imminent surgery.

For total cure the homeopathic treatment must be taken seriously for about 12 to 18 months depending upon the number and size of uterine fibroids or myomas.

Naturopathy and fibroids

Naturopathy is a type of alternative medicine that emphasises a sensible diet, avoidance of toxins in the environment, regular exercise, adequate rest, and botanical remedies. These healthy lifestyle behaviours and the naturopathic approach are designed to stimulate the body's vital force and immune system to heal itself and restore the body to a natural state of heath balance. The naturopathic approach to treat fibroids includes:

Achieving and maintaining a weight-to-height ratio that is not considered overweight

Avoiding caffeine-containing foods and beverages

Avoiding excessive consumption of alcoholic beverages

Eating a diet that limits the amount of oestrogen consumed from animal products, tends to counteracts oestrogen dominance (i.e. counteracts a higher ratio of levels of oestrogen to levels of androgen such as progesterone) in the body, and /or tends to have anti-oestrogen effects

Taking supplements that counteract oestrogen dominance and /or have anti-oestrogen effects. Examples are supplements containing chaste tree berries, diindolylmethane (DIM), flavinoids, flaxseeds or flaxseed oil, lady's mantle, lipotropic factors, saw palmetto, and yarrow flowers.

Taking supplements such as thyroid glandular extracts to help improve the function of a diagnosed under-active thyroid gland.

Taking herbal supplements to maintain health of the liver, whose role is to detoxify the body. Examples are supplements containing artichoke leaf, barberry, choline dandelion root, goldenseal, inositol, lecithin, lipotropic factors (which help break down fat and oestrogen, methionine, S-adenosyl methionine, and silymarin.

Taking herbal supplements to help stimulate blood flow to the pelvis. Herbal ingredients for this purpose include cayenne pepper and the Chinese combination herbal preparation, Bupleurum Entangled Qi Formula. Consult your integrative medical physician for guidance on the dose and supplement that is appropriate for you.

Taking supplements to help the function of the immune system and maintain uterine health. Examples of supplements are aginine, coenzyme Q10, lysine, malate mushrooms, vitamin A, vitamin C, and zinc.

Taking supplements that have anti-inflammatory activity and/or anti-oxidant activity. Examples of supplements are those containing beta-carotene, borage oil, evening primrose oil (which contains gamma linoleic acid) selenium, vitamin C, and vitamin E.

Taking supplements that can detoxify the body by helping eliminate heavy metals. Examples of supplements are systeine, glutathione, kelp, and selenium.

Taking supplements such as Calcium and magnesium to prevent and reduce muscle cramps.

Taking supplements such as kelp that can reduce the severity of fibroids and aid in healing from fibroids

Taking supplements that can help break down fibroids. Example of supplements are pancreatic enzymes and proteolytic enzymes.

Applying warm packs of castor oil to the skin over the fibroid when you are experiencing pain from the fibroid.

Taking prescription (natural or synthetic) thyroid hormone (i.e. thyroxin) if you have been diagnosed as being hypothyroid (i.e. having an under-active or inactive thyroid gland)

Using natural progesterone cream for pre-menopausal women with fibroids and post-menopausal women with fibroids. For pre-menopausal women with fibroids, the cream is applied except when menstruating. Consult your integrative medical physician for guidance on the dose that is appropriate for you.

Avoiding smoking

Avoiding exposure to environmental toxins, including cigarette smoke from other people

Regularly exercising for a minimum of 20 minutes per session, performed at least 3 times per week

Doing daily or every-other-day exercise (such as certain yoga routines) that involve movement of the pelvis, to enhance blood flow to and removal of toxins from the pelvic region

Having acupuncture for correcting energy flow and reducing pain

Stress reduction and relaxation methods, including meditation

Exploring creative endeavours

Doing other activities that are healthy, give you pleasure and make you happy

Building and maintaining good relationships with a romantic partner, family, friends, and work colleagues

Having an active and fulfilling sex life

Personally evaluating both any situations that may be resulting in powerful negative emotions, such as frustration, anxiety and stress. Working with a psychologist can help you to examine your life, modify undesirable situations, and change your feelings

Practising visualization techniques to help shrink the fibroid
Practicing prayer to help shrink the fibroid

Yoga exercises for fibroids

Yoga can tone the uterus, giving it the required strength to reduce the size and occurrence of fibroids. It is generally safe for women with fibroids, but if you have additional medical conditions such as spinal disease, high blood pressure, glaucoma, ear problems or a risk of blood clots, check with your doctor before starting a yoga program.

Bharadvaja's Twist

If you have uterine fibroids, focus on opening and softening the abdominal area to help the body accommodate fibroid growth by practising twists like Bharadvaja's Twist. To perform the twist, begin seated on your mat with your legs extended straight in front of you. Shift your weight to the right, bend your knees and then swing your legs to the left, drawing the feet toward and behind your buttocks. Breathe into the twist by inhaling, lifting through the chest and then exhaling as you twist first your torso gently to the right. Turn the neck and then the face to the right, lengthening the spine and continually breathing and lifting through the chest to intensify the twist.

Reclining Bound Angle Pose

If you experience heavy menstrual periods and pain as part of your fibroid symptoms, a restorative practice –

similar to the ones used by pregnant women to help ease discomfort and further open the abdomen – might help. To perform Reclining Bound Angle Pose, begin by sitting on your mat with knees bent out to the sides and the soles of your feet touching. Place thick blankets on either side of your hips to support your thighs and bring greater ease to this restorative posture. Next, use your hands to support yourself as you lean back and then lie flat on the floor, keeping your knees bent outward and resting your bent knees on the blankets. Close your eyes, breathe deeply and focus on sending your groins deep down into your pelvis, widening the back pelvis and narrowing the front. Allow the knees to slowly and naturally move closer to the floor as you focus on your groins. Do not push the knees down actively.

Supported Bridge Pose

To perform the supported version of Bridge Pose, keep a block or bolster by your mat as you lie down on your back and bend your knees, drawing the feet as close to the buttocks as possible and keeping the arms straight at your sides. Exhale and push your tailbone up while pressing your feet firmly into the floor, lifting your buttocks off the ground and supporting yourself by placing the block or bolster beneath your sacrum. Draw your shoulder blades together and down your back, and maintain active thighs and arms for additional support.

Reclining hero pose

If you have uterine fibroids, you might also want to try Reclining Hero Pose.

However, it is important to note that this pose is an intermediate yoga posture and should only be practiced if you can already perform Hero Pose, a seated posture in which the buttocks sits on the floor between the feet, with relative ease. To transition from Hero Pose to Reclining Hero Pose, exhale and slowly lower your back toward the floor, using your hands and arms for support. If needed, place blankets beneath your back for added cushion and ease. Lay your arms on the floor slightly away from your body, with the palms facing upward. Keep the thighs parallel and the knees as parallel as possible. Do not allow the knees to fall any wider apart than hip's width to prevent strain.

Acupuncture for fibroids

Acupuncture is widely known to be highly effective at relieving the symptoms of fibroids. "Used regularly, acupuncture can help to prevent fibroids developing" says Maureen Cromey, a registered member of the British Acupuncture Council. "In Chinese medical theory, fibroids are considered to be caused by stagnant blood forming masses in and around the womb. Acupuncture helps by improving circulation of qi and blood in the area, relieving symptoms such as pain and bleeding, as well as reducing the size of fibroids.

Reflexology for fibroids

Reflexology can also help as research studies have shown it can reduce pain. "Reflexologists believe there is balancing of the hormonal system and an increase in circulation as a result of a reflexology treatment," says Tracey Smith of the Association of Reflexologists. "Treatment can also help to relieve stress and tension and aims to help the body to do what it wants to do, which is heal."

The list of alternative and natural therapies that are helpful for fibroid sufferers is exhaustive and the above therapies and exercises are just a very small example as to what is available and very beneficial for fibroid sufferers. It pays to browse the web at your own leisure so that you can decide on what might be the best and most suitable treatment for yourself. Whether it is offered freely through the NHS, by your doctor or privately, you should be able to access the right treatment that feels right for you and that which appeals to you most and one that is most beneficial for your own individual need.

CHAPTER 4

The emotional factor and its contribution to the development of fibroids

Most conventional doctors will patiently explain that the causes of fibroids are unknown. However, there is increasing evidence that emotional state may have a significant role in the development of fibroids. Several uniquely female issues or traumas have been identified as being linked to fibroids and it is not just my belief alone that emotional issues, at least in part lie behind the development of fibroids. Many practitioners in the medical arena, have and are beginning to recognise that there is indeed an emotional link to fibroids.

There is another effective way to tackle fibroids and that does not have to mean precluding any other fibroid treatment. According to theory, tackling fibroids at the emotional level means that as the issues are resolved, the underlying emotional cause of the fibroids is therefore removed and the fibroid simply dissolves away. For those who understand and accept the concept of the mind-body link, this approach is likely to resonate quite strongly and will feel naturally right.

Unresolved emotional issues can contribute to Illness

I am sure you will agree, that emotions are powerful. Think of how your body feels when you are happy or sad. Chinese Medical theory states that emotions alone can cause dis-ease in the body. When it comes to uterine fibroids, this is no exception.

There is much research about surgical or drug therapy for the treatment of fibroids, adequate information about diet and far less about the emotional aspects of fibroids. There is much documentation however, about the relationship between myomas and stuck energy/emotions and the importance of working with and releasing energy blockages in the pelvis.

In Chinese medicine, fibroids are viewed as blood stagnation which herbs and acupuncture can begin moving. However, stagnation of the blood is preceded by stagnant energy, i.e. emotions. Thus therapies work best when a patient is proactive and does personal emotional work. Emotional issues can affect your biology in profound and often undesirable ways. Unresolved emotional issues are often associated with gynaecological problems such as uterine fibroids, ovarian cysts, and excessive bleeding is according to some alternative practitioners, the body's need to express itself.

One wise doctor was reported as saying and concerning this subject of the body's need to express itself that "If you don't cry above, you'll cry below." The crying below refers to the uterus, whose "tears" are menstrual blood. Strong emotions, if left unaddressed, will manifest themselves as body symptoms, such as excessive menstrual bleeding. The body is always metaphorical and listens to the psyche of the individual and responds accordingly in its own way, translating withheld tears into copious menstrual flow. The emotional issue is an energy that has to go somewhere; it has to be expressed physiologically. For example, if we look at the subject of unexpressed anger; we do carry a lot of emotions and experiences in our wombs and the inability to eliminate those emotional toxins (like physical toxins and chemicals) will cause disease. Fibroids basically are housing a mixture of physical toxins and emotional toxins that the body is attempting to wall off, but eventually get so big that they cause complications! Some alternative therapists consider the womb to be the creative seat of women and thus the seat of a woman's power! In the course of life we can often get caught in a rut/environment that is non-conducive to our creative side and this causes stagnation in our centre of energy, which is why many women with fibroids usually have other issues aside from just the gynaecological symptoms, i.e. depression, anxiety, fear, abuse, feeling unfulfilled, toxic relationships etc. Sometimes these "other issues" can be the root causes of the dis-ease in the first place, with the fibroid (and other symptoms) just being a physical manifestation of everything going on. It is my own personal belief, as a holistic therapist and counsellor, that emotional toxins can be just as detrimental as physical toxins. As multifaceted beings, an approach that addresses ALL of us – mental, physical and emotional (not forgetting the spiritual) should be implemented in each of our lives in order that true healing can occur.

Stress Reduction For Relief of Fibroids

Fibroids as we have seen can be caused or exacerbated by stress. One simple exercise in combating stress and its harmful effects is to learn to control and slow down your breathing during times of stress. Lie in a quiet room where you are unlikely to be disturbed. Place one hand on your abdomen and the other on your upper chest. Take a slow, deep breath in through your mouth, making sure it bypasses the upper hand so that it reaches the lower hand on your upper abdomen. Hold the breath for a few seconds and slowly release the breath out through your mouth in a controlled way. Wait a couple of seconds before repeating the process. Initially only practice this for five breaths, as any more may leave you feeling lightheaded.

Looking at the triggers and more helpful techniques and exercises for the treatment and prevention of fibroids

Emotional injuries, suppression of creativity and other factors can contribute to the growth of problematic fibroid tumours. For example:

Relationship Trauma
Termination or Miscarriage
Sexual Abuse in Formative years
Difficult Childhoods
Taking Care of others in a negative, co-dependency situation
Giving up on dreams
Strict Religious upbringing

According to author, Debbie Shapiro (author of 'Your body Speaks Your Mind') says fibroids are a gathering of mental patterns or attitudes that have been suppressed for so long that they have taken a solid form. Uterine fibroids are connected to our feelings of femininity, sexuality, womanhood or motherhood. "There may be accumulated or unexpressed guilt, shame, loss grief, inner confusion or past hurt and abuse."

Finding the trigger

When looking for the root to any emotional or physical problem and as in this case, fibroids, you might ask yourself a series of questions:

When did you first notice the symptoms?
What was happening in your life just before that? What was bothering you? What changes were going on? (The majority of people just "know" what triggered their illness when asked.)
How did that make you feel? (E.g. Sad, lonely, criticised, abandoned, helpless,

frightened, guilty, furious, invisible, inadequate, ashamed, unloved, disappointed, frustrated, resentful, betrayed, bewildered, unwanted, confused)?

When was the earliest time you remember feeling that way?

What negative belief or decision arose from that experience (eg. I am not safe in the world. Men abandon me. I am not good enough. I must hide my feelings.)? If you are not sure, just take a guess. Or imagine that you are talking to that part of you that you don't know.

Once you know what triggered the problem, you can start to tackle it by writing about it in a journal, writing an imaginary letter to the person involved then burning it, and using various forms of psychological exercise therapy. Below are a few suggestions to help you on your journey.

Write. Writing can release explore, and express. Write letters to your womb or from your womb to yourself. Allow yourself to feel the emotions that surface and cry or rant – whatever comes up.

Let go. Are you holding onto painful past experiences? Do you experience unresolved anger, fear, lack of self love, guilt, blame? Traumatic experiences can be difficult to deal with. Talk to a therapist, or someone you can trust. Work to learn how to stop suppressing them.

Visualise. Visualization techniques use images you can create in your mind to bring about physiological changes in your body. One visualization exercise for fibroids uses an 'erasure' image that helps you see your fibroids melt away and disappear.

Sit in a comfortable position. Close your eyes. Begin to breathe deeply. Inhale and let the air out slowly. Feel your body begin to relax.

Imagine that you can look, as if through a magic mirror, deep inside your own body.

Now look at your female organs. See your uterus and ovaries. They are an attractive pink colour. Your uterus is relaxed and supple. Any fibroid tumours are melting away as you look at them. Your uterus is becoming its normal size and shape. Your uterus has good blood circulation. Look at your ovaries. They are extremely healthy and put out just the right levels of hormones. They are shiny and pink and look like two little almonds. The fallopian tubes that pick up the eggs and bring them to the uterus are totally open and healthy.

Look at your abdominal wall and low back muscles. They are soft and pliable with a healthy muscle tone. They are relaxed and free of tension during your menstrual period. Your abdomen is flat and your fluid balance is perfect in your pelvic area.

Look at your entire body and enjoy the sense of peace and calm running through your body. You feel wonderful.

Stop visualizing the scene, and focus on your deep breathing, inhaling and exhaling slowly.

You open your eyes and feel very good. Visualizing this scene should take a minute or two. Linger on any images that particularly please you.

Make positive affirmations about how you want your body to be.

Fibroids can be aggravated by negative thoughts because when your body believes it is sick then it behaves accordingly. It is therefore, essential as part of your healing program to have and cultivate a positive body image. Making positive affirmations is a very simple technique that can be practised anywhere and it involves the power of suggestion. All that is involved is the repetition, aloud or mentally of a certain phrase. You can sit in a comfortable position and repeat each affirmation below three times:

My female system is strong and healthy
My hormonal levels are perfectly balanced and regulated.

My body chemistry is healthy and balanced.

I go through my monthly menstrual cycle with ease and comfort.

My menstrual flow self-regulates.

I have light to moderate bleeding.

My body is relaxed and pain-free.

My vaginal muscles are relaxed and comfortable.

My cervix and uterus are relaxed and pain-free.

My uterus is normal in size and shape.

My menstrual flow leaves my body easily and effortlessly each month.

My body feels wonderful as I start each monthly period.

I barely know that my body is getting ready to menstruate.

I feel wonderful each month before I menstruate.

My uterus is relaxed and receptive; I welcome my monthly period.

My low back muscles feel supple and pliable with each menstrual cycle.

I am relaxed and at ease as my period approaches.

I desire a well balanced and healthful diet.

I eat only the foods that are good for my female body.

It is a real pleasure to take good care of my body.

I do the level of exercise that keeps my body healthy and supple.

I handle stress easily and in a relaxed manner.

I love my body; I feel at ease in my body.

My body is pain-free and relaxed.

Gradually, these affirmations will become a sort of background music to your life, always ticking over in your mind, no matter where you are or what you are doing. You will find that you come to believe what you are saying and that, after all, is what it is all about.

Clear away unhealthy relationships. Learn how to recognize relationships that do not serve. Putting energy into a dead end relationship or job is feeding your fibroids. Know that there is no one way or path. There are options, the choice is yours.

Express yourself. It has been recognised that fibroids are the result of unexpressed creativity and unrealized self-expression. How are you holding yourself back?

Listen to your body

In her book, "Cure fibroids naturally", Gillian Bowles says, "Take responsibility for yourself, take back your own power and listen to your body. You have all you need within. Learn a new way with regard to taking care of your health and your body. Start to develop your spiritual side. You already know some of the things you need to do to lead a healthier life, make it as much fun as you can. Take time out to do things you love, some of which you may not have done for years."

I wish you well, on your journey to a much healthier you. God bless you and thank you for reading!

www.ingramcontent.com/pod-product-compliance
Lightning Source LLC
Chambersburg PA
CBHW060431290526
45791CB00002B/922